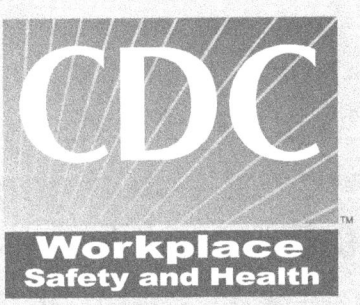

Crystalline Silica and Isocyanate Exposures during Parking Garage Repair

Chandran Achutan, PhD

Ayodele Adebayo, MD, MPH

Fariba Nourian, BS

Health Hazard Evaluation Report
HETA 2008-0058-3108
Aduddell Restoration and Waterproofing, Inc.
Arlington, Virginia
April 2010

Department of Health and Human Services
Centers for Disease Control and Prevention

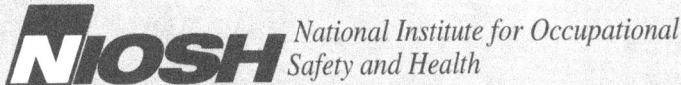

National Institute for Occupational Safety and Health

The employer shall post a copy of this report for a period of 30 calendar days at or near the workplace(s) of affected employees. The employer shall take steps to insure that the posted determinations are not altered, defaced, or covered by other material during such period. [37 FR 23640, November 7, 1972, as amended at 45 FR 2653, January 14, 1980].

CONTENTS

ABBREVIATIONS

µg/m³	Micrograms per cubic meter
µm	Micrometer
ACGIH®	American Conference of Governmental Industrial Hygienists
CFR	Code of Federal Regulations
HHE	Health hazard evaluation
IARC	International Agency for Research on Cancer
Lpm	Liters per minute
mg/m³	Milligrams per cubic meter
mm	Millimeter
mppcf	Million particles per cubic foot
MDI	Methylenebis(phenyl isocyanate)
MSDS	Material safety data sheet
NAICS	North American Industry Classification System
NIOSH	National Institute for Occupational Safety and Health
OEL	Occupational exposure limit
OSHA	Occupational Safety and Health Administration
PBZ	Personal breathing zone
PPE	Personal protective equipment
PEL	Permissible exposure limit
REL	Recommended exposure limit
STEL	Short-term exposure limit
TLV®	Threshold limit value
TRIG	Total reactive isocyanate group
TWA	Time-weighted average
UK HSE	United Kingdom Health and Safety Executive
WEEL	Workplace environmental exposure limit

The National Institute for Occupational Safety and Health (NIOSH) received a management request for a health hazard evaluation at Aduddell Restoration and Waterproofing, Inc. in Arlington, Virginia. The request was submitted because management wanted to ensure that employees were adequately protected against silica and methylenebis(phenyl isocyanate) exposure (MDI).

What NIOSH Did

- We evaluated the worksite in January and February 2008.
- We talked to all employees at the site about their health concerns.
- We measured airborne dust and crystalline silica.
- We analyzed samples of filler Part A and Part B for MDI monomer.
- We tested how long it takes for MDI-containing Part A and castor oil-containing Part B to react with each other.

What NIOSH Found

- No employees at the site reported work-related health concerns.
- Employees were overexposed to crystalline silica while jackhammering and sandblasting.
- Filler Part A contained 52% MDI monomer. Part B contained no MDI monomer.
- Unreacted MDI monomer was present for at least 40 minutes after employees mixed Parts A and B mixed together, causing potential dermal exposure for employees.
- Employees wore respirators when jackhammering, sandblasting, and mixing Parts A and B, but not when applying filler material.
- Employees were not respirator fit-tested.
- Employees did not clean or maintain their respirators properly.
- Employees who used the jack hammer wore leather gloves instead of antivibration gloves.
- Some employees did not wear eye protection while sandblasting, jackhammering, or mixing and applying filler material.
- Noise levels during jackhammering and sandblasting need evaluation. A hearing conservation program may be warranted.

What Managers Can Do

- Require employees to wear respirators while jackhammering and sandblasting.

- Require employees to wear eye protection while sandblasting, jackhammering, or mixing and applying filler material.

- Comply with the Occupational Safety and Health Administration (OSHA) Respiratory Protection Standard. This standard includes elements of training, correct use and maintenance, and fit testing of respirators.

- Explore possible engineering controls to reduce dust levels while jackhammering and sandblasting.

- Comply with the OSHA Hazard Communication Standard. Provide training on all hazards such as silica, isocyanates, and vibration.

- Evaluate employees' noise exposure during jackhammering and sandblasting.

- Provide employees who use vibrating tools, such as jackhammers, with antivibration gloves.

- Provide employees who work with Part A and the mixed compound with butyl rubber gloves.

- Establish a smoking cessation program and encourage employees to use it to quit smoking.

What Employees Can Do

- Continue to wear respirators while jackhammering and sandblasting.

- Clean and store your respirator at the end of the work day.

- Be clean shaven so the respirator fits properly.

- Wear antivibration gloves when jackhammering.

- Wear butyl rubber gloves when handling Part A and the Part A and B mixture.

- Wear eye protection while sandblasting, jackhammering, or mixing and applying filler material.

- Stop smoking.

On November 30, 2007, NIOSH received a request from managers at Aduddell Restoration and Waterproofing, Inc. for an HHE at the Ballston Mall Parking Garage in Arlington, Virginia. The managers wanted to know if the employees were adequately protected against silica and MDI during parking garage repair.

Full-shift PBZ air samples for respirable particulates and silica were collected on four employees over 2 days. The amount of MDI monomer in a bulk sample of Part A and Part B was measured. We also evaluated the curing time after mixing MDI-containing Part A and the inert Part B.

Employees were exposed to hazardous levels of respirable crystalline silica during jackhammering and sandblasting. Of the eight PBZ air samples for respirable dust and silica, seven reached or exceeded the silica (as quartz) ACGIH TLV of 0.025 mg/m³, and six reached or exceeded the NIOSH REL of 0.05 mg/m³. None of the samples exceeded the OSHA Construction PEL for respirable dust containing silica (quartz). Approximately 52% of the bulk sample of Part A was MDI monomer. Part B contained no MDI monomer. A quantitative analysis of the reaction between Part A and Part B showed that approximately 80% of the MDI monomer reacted in the first 10 minutes. At 60 minutes, the mixture was hardened. We considered inhalation exposure to MDI unlikely because of the low vapor pressure of MDI, the relatively short curing time between the MDI-containing Part A and the inert Part B, and the method used to pour and apply the MDI-containing slurry. However, we believed there was a potential for dermal exposure to MDI that could result in sensitization, asthma, and contact dermatitis.

We interviewed all 10 employees who were working during our site visit; none reported work-related health concerns. The company provided the appropriate type of respirator for crystalline silica and required employees to wear it. However, not all job tasks requiring respirators were clearly defined. Additionally, employees were neither respirator fit-tested nor did they clean or maintain their respirators properly.

We recommend informing employees that MDI monomer may still exist after Parts A and B are mixed together and requiring them to wear butyl rubber gloves when mixing these compounds. We also recommend requiring employees to wear respirators during jackhammering and sandblasting. The company's respirator program should comply with the OSHA Respiratory

Employees were overexposed to crystalline silica when jackhammering and sandblasting. Employees may be exposed to MDI through skin contact and should wear butyl rubber gloves to minimize exposure. Although the appropriate respirator was available for crystalline silica exposure, not all job tasks requiring respirators were clearly identified in the company's respirator program.

Protection Standard. Additional recommendations included exploring possible engineering controls to reduce dust levels while jackhammering and sandblasting; complying with the OSHA Hazard Communication Standard; evaluating employees' exposure to noise during jackhammering and sandblasting activities; providing antivibration gloves to employees who use vibrating tools such as jackhammers; wearing eye protection while sandblasting, jackhammering, or mixing and applying filler material; and establishing a smoking cessation program.

Keywords: NAICS 238390 (Other Building Finishing Contractors), respirable dust, silica, quartz, isocyanate, MDI, curing time

INTRODUCTION

On November 30, 2007, NIOSH received a request from the management of Aduddell Restoration and Waterproofing, Inc. (Aduddell) for an HHE at the Ballston Mall Parking Garage in Arlington, Virginia. Aduddell is based in Minneapolis, Minnesota, but carries out contract work across the country. Managers at Aduddell wanted to know if their employees were adequately protected against silica and MDI during parking garage repair.

On January 12–14, 2008, and February 13–14, 2008, NIOSH investigators visited the Ballston Mall Parking Garage in Arlington, Virginia, to evaluate employee exposure to respirable silica and MDI. During both visits, employees were repairing the first and second floors of the parking garage. Areas needing minor repairs are first prepped by applying MDI-containing slurry as a filler material. Employees remove damaged concrete by jackhammering and sandblasting continuously for a few hours or sporadically throughout the day. Employees prepare the filler material by mixing one part of Part A, an MDI-containing product, and two parts of Part B, containing primarily castor oil, in a bucket. Sand is added to the mixture to make it easier to spread. The entire mixing process takes about 30 seconds.

ASSESSMENT

To determine the presence of potential work-related health effects, employees were asked to describe any health problems that they were experiencing including those they attributed to work exposures. We interviewed all 10 employees present in a private setting.

We collected full-shift PBZ air samples for respirable particulates from four employees jackhammering and sandblasting over 2 days. The samples were collected and analyzed according to NIOSH Method 0600 [NIOSH 2009]. Samples were collected on 37-mm, 5-µm polyvinyl chloride filters, at a flow rate of 1.7 Lpm using a 10-mm nylon cyclone preselector for respirable particulate. The respirable particulate samples were also analyzed for silica content by x-ray diffraction with NIOSH Method 7500 [NIOSH 2009].

According to the MSDS, the active ingredient in Part A is 25%–70% MDI monomer, and the active ingredient in Part B is 60%–100% castor oil. Bulk samples of Parts A and B were collected and analyzed for MDI monomer in accordance with NIOSH Method 5525 [NIOSH 2009]. Managers assumed that once Parts A and B were mixed in the bucket the reaction was complete and that MDI monomer, the active ingredient that can potentially cause adverse health effects, no longer existed. To test this assumption, we studied the reaction that occurs between Parts A and B over time. To accomplish this, we mixed one part of Part A and two parts of Part B in six vials and allowed them to react for 5, 10, 15, 20, 40, or 60 minutes. The reactions were halted at these time intervals by diluting the reaction solutions and analyzing for MDI monomer according to NIOSH Method 5525 [NIOSH 2009].

For information on the OELs and health effects of silica and isocyanates (including MDI), please see Appendix A.

RESULTS

Employee Interviews

All interviewed employees were men who had worked for Aduddell from 2 months to 17 years. Only three of the employees had worked at the company for more than a year. Four employees reported ever working with Part A. None of the 10 employees reported adverse health symptoms or work-related health problems. All the employees reported that hard hats and safety shoes were mandatory during work, while respirators, earplugs, safety glasses, and leather or rubber gloves were used when deemed necessary by the employer. Employees reported that they had not been fit-tested for respirator use.

Respirable Dust and Silica

All of the crystalline silica in the respirable dust samples was present as quartz. As summarized in Table 1, of the eight respirable dust and quartz PBZ air samples, seven reached or exceeded the quartz ACGIH TLV of 0.025 mg/m³ [ACGIH 2009], and six reached or exceeded the NIOSH REL of 0.05 mg/m³ [NIOSH 2005]. None of the samples exceeded the OSHA Construction PEL for respirable dust containing silica (quartz) (refer to Appendix A for a description on how to calculate the PEL) [29 CFR 1910.1000].

Table 1. Full-shift PBZ respirable dust and respirable silica (as quartz) exposures during jack hammering and sandblasting

Employee	Sampling Time (min)	Respirable Dust (mg/m³)	Respirable Dust 8-hr (mg/m³)	Respirable Dust (mppcf)	Respirable Dust 8-hr (mppcf)	Respirable Quartz (mg/m³)	Respirable Quartz 8-hr (mg/m³)	Quartz (%)	OSHA PEL* (mppcf)
				2/13/08					
1	323	0.67	0.45	6.7	4.5	0.15	0.10	21.6	9.4
2	305	0.65	0.41	6.5	4.1	0.13	0.08	19.4	10
3	309	0.25	0.16	2.5	1.6	0.05	0.03	21.5	9.4
4	297	1.3	0.78	13	7.8	0.22	0.13	17.2	11
				2/14/08					
1	349	0.23	0.17	2.3	1.7	0.04	0.03	16.4	12
2	346	0.56	0.40	5.6	4.0	0.08	0.06	14.9	13
3	348	0.42	0.31	4.2	4.2	0.07	0.05	17.2	11
4	347	0.25	0.18	2.5	2.5	0.02	0.01	7.3	20
NIOSH REL						0.05	0.05		
ACGIH TLV						0.025	0.025		

*OSHA Construction PEL for respirable dust containing silica (quartz)

Methylenebis(phenyl isocyanate)

Analysis of a Part A bulk sample showed that it contained approximately 52% MDI monomer, while the analysis of Part B did not detect MDI monomer. Quantitative analysis of the reaction between Part A and Part B showed that approximately 80% of the MDI monomer reacted in the first 10 minutes. The mixture was completely hardened at 60 minutes and therefore could not be analyzed for MDI. Figure 1 shows the curing time following mixing of Parts A and B.

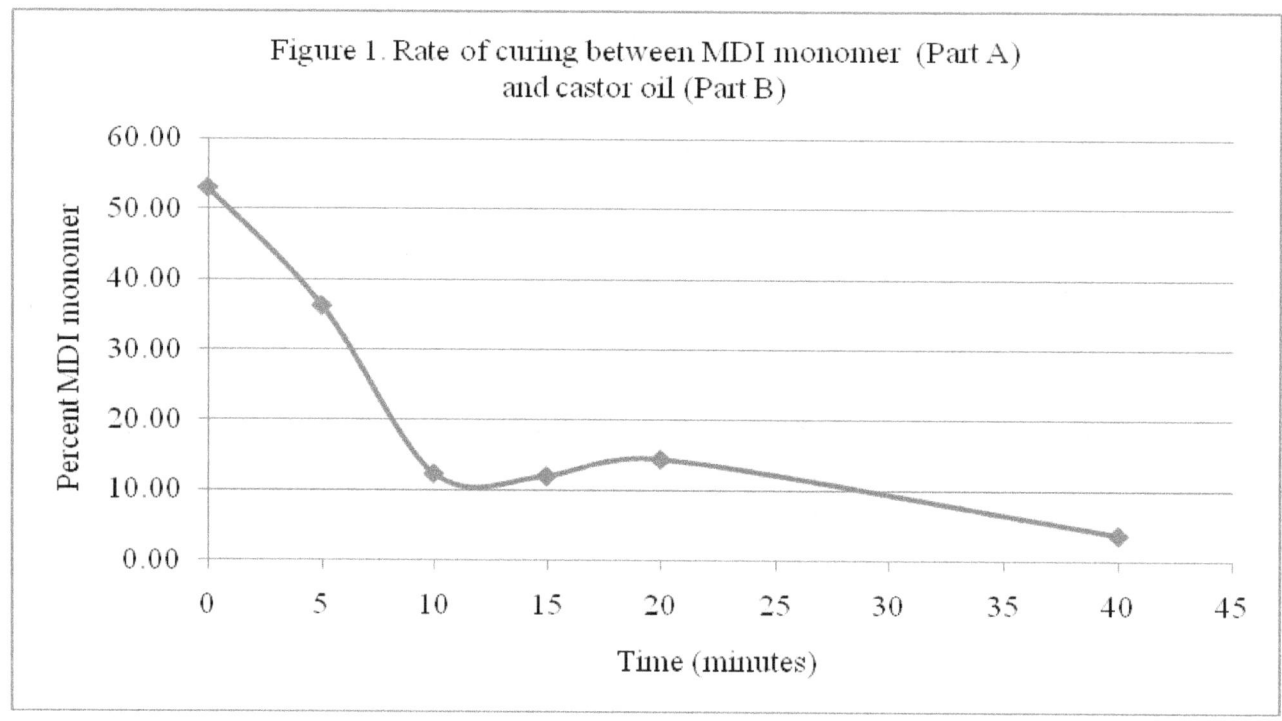

Figure 1. Rate of curing between MDI monomer (Part A) and castor oil (Part B)

Other Observations

Employees were wearing respirators during jackhammering, sandblasting, and the mixing of Parts A and B, but not during the filler material application. Although Aduddell had a written respiratory protection program, the job tasks requiring respirators were not clearly identified. Employees were not respirator fit-tested and did not clean or maintain their respirators properly.

All the employees performed their tasks in street clothes without a set of clean clothes for changing after work. Some employees wore no eye protection while sandblasting, jackhammering, or mixing and applying filler material. We noted that employees used leather gloves for jackhammering instead of antivibration gloves. Employees were smoking in the workplace without first washing their hands. Although noise exposures were not part of this HHE and were not evaluated, our opinion is that the noise generated by jackhammering and sandblasting activities may exceed OELs and warrant future evaluation.

DISCUSSION

The results from the particulate sampling showed that employees were overexposed to crystalline silica. However, employees were wearing NIOSH-certified, air-purifying elastomeric half-mask respirators equipped with P100 particulate filters. These respirators can protect them from crystalline silica exposure if worn properly within the context of a complete respirator program. A complete program requires that respirator wearers are clean-shaven, fit-tested, and medically cleared to wear a respirator and that respirators are cleaned and maintained properly. Additionally, to avoid confusion, Aduddell's respirator program should clearly identify the activities where respirator use is required. Implementing engineering or administrative controls to reduce employee exposures to silica-containing dust generated by jackhammering and sandblasting could reduce or eliminate the need for respirator use. The OSHA website at http://www.osha.gov/SLTC/silicacrystalline/index.html and NIOSH website at http://www.cdc.gov/niosh/topics/silica/ provide information on engineering and administrative controls that may be useful to Aduddell in reducing employee exposures.

The low vapor pressure of MDI, the relatively short curing time between the MDI-containing Part A and the inert Part B, and the pour-application method of the MDI-containing slurry (as opposed to spray application), makes it unlikely that employees applying the slurry were overexposed to airborne MDI. However, there is a potential for dermal exposure among these employees. Skin sensitization to MDI is possible, and if skin sensitization were to occur, employees would not be able to work around MDI-containing substances without serious medical problems, such as dermatitis or asthma. Employees were under the impression that after they mixed Parts A and B, the resulting mixture was inert. Although 80% of the MDI monomer reacted in the first 10 minutes, our reaction time study shows that the reaction goes on for at least 40 minutes. Additionally, employees smoking in the workplace without first washing their hands can increase MDI exposure by ingesting chemicals from hand to mouth.

Jackhammering, sandblasting, and preparing and applying the filler material all have the potential to create an eye hazard. Using goggles or safety glasses while conducting these tasks can reduce the possibility of eye injuries. Additional information is available at http://www.cdc.gov/niosh/topics/eye/.

CONCLUSIONS

Although employees reported no health concerns, they were overexposed to respirable crystalline silica during jackhammering and sandblasting. Inhalation exposure to MDI appears unlikely; however, there was a potential for dermal exposure to MDI, which can cause sensitization to isocyanates and put employees at risk for dermatitis and asthma.

RECOMMENDATIONS

Based on our findings, we recommend the actions listed below to create a more healthful workplace. We encourage Aduddell to use a labor-management health and safety committee or working group to discuss the recommendations in this report and develop an action plan. Those involved in the work can best set priorities and assess the feasibility of our recommendations for the specific situation at Aduddell. Our recommendations are based on the hierarchy of controls approach (refer to Appendix A: Occupational Exposure Limits and Health Effects). This approach groups actions by their likely effectiveness in reducing or removing hazards. In most cases, the preferred approach is to eliminate hazardous materials or processes and install engineering controls to reduce exposure or shield employees. Until such controls are in place, or if they are not effective or feasible, administrative measures and/or personal protective equipment may be needed.

Engineering Controls

Engineering controls reduce exposures to employees by removing the hazard from the process or placing a barrier between the hazard and the employee. Engineering controls are very effective at protecting employees without placing primary responsibility of implementation on the employee.

1. Reduce dust levels while jackhammering and sandblasting by exhausting the dust close to its point of production. Links for information on engineering controls are available at http://www.cdc.gov/niosh/topics/silica/.

Administrative Controls

Administrative controls are management-dictated work practices and policies to reduce or prevent exposures to workplace hazards.

Recommendations

The effectiveness of administrative changes in work practices for controlling workplace hazards is dependent on management commitment and employee acceptance. Regular monitoring and reinforcement are necessary to ensure that control policies and procedures are not circumvented in the name of convenience or production.

1. Ensure that requirements listed in the OSHA Respiratory Protection Standard [29 CFR 1910.134] are established in Aduddell's written program and are followed. Ensure that employees are medically cleared, fit-tested, clean-shaven, and adequately trained on respirator use and care before they use respirators. Additional respirator use information is available at http://www.osha.gov/SLTC/etools/silica/index.html and http://www.osha.gov/Publications/SECG_RPS/secg_rps.html.

2. Update the current respiratory protection program to reflect the job tasks requiring the use of a respirator and the type of respirator to be worn.

3. Educate employees on the health effects and proper work practices when working with crystalline silica, isocyanates, and vibration as required by the OSHA Hazard Communication Standard [29 CFR 1910.1200]. Make them aware that MDI monomer may still be present even after Parts A and B are mixed together. Additional hazard communication information is available at http://www.osha.gov/dsg/hazcom/index.html.

4. Evaluate employee noise exposures and, if needed, establish a hearing conservation program. The basic elements of the program should meet, at a minimum, the requirements of the OSHA hearing conservation amendment [29 CFR 1910.95]. Other sources for defining effective hearing conservation programs are also available [Royster and Royster 1990; NIOSH 1996; Suter 2002].

5. Establish a smoking cessation program and encourage employees to use it to quit smoking. MDI from their hands could be transferred onto the cigarettes, and this could lead to respiratory exposure. In addition, tobacco products have been shown to cause many adverse health effects including respiratory diseases and cancer. Further information regarding workplace smoking policies and smoking cessation programs can be found in (1) *NIOSH Current Intelligence Bulletin 54: Environmental Tobacco Smoke in the Workplace,*

Lung Cancer and Other Health Effects, (2) *The Health Consequences of Smoking: a Report of the Surgeon General*, and (3) *Environmental Tobacco Smoke* [NIOSH 1991; DHHS 2004; ASHRAE 2005].

Personal Protective Equipment

PPE is the least effective means for controlling employee exposures. Proper use of PPE requires a comprehensive program and calls for a high level of employee involvement and commitment to be effective. The use of PPE requires the choice of the appropriate equipment to reduce the hazard and the development of supporting programs such as training, change-out schedules, and medical assessment if needed. PPE should not be relied upon as the sole method for limiting employee exposures. Rather, PPE should be used until engineering and administrative controls can be demonstrated to be effective in limiting exposures to acceptable levels.

1. Continue to use the respirators currently provided to employees until engineering or administrative controls can be implemented to reduce crystalline silica exposures to below the OELs.

2. Employees should have separate work clothes or clean sets of clothes at the worksite. This will allow them to change to clean clothes if they spill MDI-containing products on their clothing.

3. Employees should wear goggles and butyl rubber gloves when mixing filler material Parts A and B.

4. Ensure that employees jackhammering and sandblasting wear eye protection, and provide antivibration gloves to employees who work with jackhammers. Hearing protection should be used if noise levels exceed OELs.

REFERENCES

ACGIH [2009]. 2009 TLVs® and BEIs®: threshold limit values for chemical substances and physical agents and biological exposure indices. Cincinnati, OH: American Conference of Governmental Industrial Hygienists.

ASHRAE [2005]. Environmental tobacco smoke: position document [http://www.ashrae.org/content/ASHRAE/ASHRAE/ArticleAltFormat/20058211239_347.pdf]. Date accessed: December 2009.

CFR. Code of Federal Regulations. Washington, DC: U.S. Government Printing Office, Office of the Federal Register.

DHHS [2004]. The health consequences of smoking: a report of the Surgeon General. Atlanta, GA: U.S. Department of Health and Human Services, Centers for Disease Control and Prevention, National Center for Chronic Disease Prevention and Health Promotion, Office on Smoking and Health.

NIOSH [1991]. Current intelligence bulletin 54: environmental tobacco smoke in the workplace, lung cancer and other health effects. By Votaw DM, Steenland K. Cincinnati, OH: U.S. Department of Health and Human Services. Centers for Disease Control, National Institute for Occupational Safety and Health, DHHS (NIOSH) Publication No. 91-108.

NIOSH [1996]. Preventing occupational hearing loss–a practical guide. By Franks JR, Stephenson MR, Merry CJ. Cincinnati, OH: U.S. Department of Health and Human Services, Centers for Disease Control and Prevention, National Institute for Occupational Safety and Health, DHHS (NIOSH) Publication No. 96-110.

NIOSH [2005]. NIOSH pocket guide to chemical hazards. Cincinnati, OH: U.S. Department of Health and Human Services, Centers for Disease Control and Prevention, National Institute for Occupational Safety and Health, DHHS (NIOSH) Publication No. 2005-149. [http://www.cdc.gov/niosh/npg/]. Date accessed: December 2009.

NIOSH [2009]. NIOSH manual of analytical methods (NMAM®). 4th ed. Schlecht PC, O'Connor PF, eds. Cincinnati, OH: U.S. Department of Health and Human Services, Centers for Disease Control and Prevention, National Institute for Occupational Safety

REFERENCES
(CONTINUED)

and Health, DHHS (NIOSH) Publication 94-113 (August, 1994); 1st Supplement Publication 96-135, 2nd Supplement Publication 98-119; 3rd Supplement 2003-154. [http://www.cdc.gov/niosh/docs/2003-154/].

Royster JD, Royster LH [1990]. Hearing conservation programs: practical guidelines for success. Chelsea, MI: Lewis Publishers.

Suter AH [2002]. Hearing conservation manual. 4th ed. Milwaukee, WI: Council for Accreditation in Occupational Hearing Conservation.

In evaluating the hazards posed by workplace exposures, NIOSH investigators use both mandatory (legally enforceable) and recommended OELs for chemical, physical, and biological agents as a guide for making recommendations. OELs have been developed by Federal agencies and safety and health organizations to prevent the occurrence of adverse health effects from workplace exposures. Generally, OELs suggest levels of exposure that most employees may be exposed up to 10 hours per day, 40 hours per week for a working lifetime without experiencing adverse health effects. However, not all employees will be protected from adverse health effects even if their exposures are maintained below these levels. A small percentage may experience adverse health effects because of individual susceptibility, a preexisting medical condition, and/or a hypersensitivity (allergy). In addition, some hazardous substances may act in combination with other workplace exposures, the general environment, or with medications or personal habits of the employee to produce health effects even if the occupational exposures are controlled at the level set by the exposure limit. Also, some substances can be absorbed by direct contact with the skin and mucous membranes in addition to being inhaled, which contributes to the individual's overall exposure.

Most OELs are expressed as a TWA exposure. A TWA refers to the average exposure during a normal 8- to 10-hour workday. Some chemical substances and physical agents have recommended STEL or ceiling values where health effects are caused by exposures over a short period. Unless otherwise noted, the STEL is a 15-minute TWA exposure that should not be exceeded at any time during a workday, and the ceiling limit is an exposure that should not be exceeded at any time.

In the United States, OELs have been established by Federal agencies, professional organizations, state and local governments, and other entities. Some OELs are legally enforceable limits, while others are recommendations. The U.S. Department of Labor OSHA PELs (29 CFR 1910 [general industry]; 29 CFR 1926 [construction industry]; and 29 CFR 1917 [maritime industry]) are legal limits enforceable in workplaces covered under the Occupational Safety and Health Act. NIOSH RELs are recommendations based on a critical review of the scientific and technical information available on a given hazard and the adequacy of methods to identify and control the hazard. NIOSH RELs can be found in the *NIOSH Pocket Guide to Chemical Hazards* [NIOSH 2005]. NIOSH also recommends different types of risk management practices (e.g., engineering controls, safe work practices, employee education/training, personal protective equipment, and exposure and medical monitoring) to minimize the risk of exposure and adverse health effects from these hazards. Other OELs that are commonly used and cited in the United States include the TLVs recommended by ACGIH, a professional organization, and the WEELs recommended by the American Industrial Hygiene Association, another professional organization. The TLVs and WEELs are developed by committee members of these associations from a review of the published, peer-reviewed literature. They are not consensus standards. ACGIH TLVs are considered voluntary exposure guidelines for use by industrial hygienists and others trained in this discipline "to assist in the control of health hazards" [ACGIH 2009]. WEELs have been established for some chemicals "when no other legal or authoritative limits exist" [AIHA 2009].

Outside the United States, OELs have been established by various agencies and organizations and include both legal and recommended limits. Since 2006, the Berufsgenossenschaftliches Institut für Arbeitsschutz (German Institute for Occupational Safety and Health) has maintained a database of international

OELs from European Union member states, Canada (Québec), Japan, Switzerland, and the United States available at http://www.dguv.de/bgia/en/gestis/limit_values/index.jsp. The database contains international limits for over 1250 hazardous substances and is updated annually.

Employers should understand that not all hazardous chemicals have specific OSHA PELs, and for some agents the legally enforceable and recommended limits may not reflect current health-based information. However, an employer is still required by OSHA to protect its employees from hazards even in the absence of a specific OSHA PEL. OSHA requires an employer to furnish employees a place of employment free from recognized hazards that cause or are likely to cause death or serious physical harm [Occupational Safety and Health Act of 1970 (Public Law 91–596, sec. 5(a)(1))]. Thus, NIOSH investigators encourage employers to make use of other OELs when making risk assessment and risk management decisions to best protect the health of their employees. NIOSH investigators also encourage the use of the traditional hierarchy of controls approach to eliminate or minimize identified workplace hazards. This includes, in order of preference, the use of: (1) substitution or elimination of the hazardous agent, (2) engineering controls (e.g , local exhaust ventilation, process enclosure, dilution ventilation), (3) administrative controls (e.g., limiting time of exposure, employee training, work practice changes, medical surveillance), and (4) personal protective equipment (e.g., respiratory protection, gloves, eye protection, hearing protection). Control banding, a qualitative risk assessment and risk management tool, is a complementary approach to protecting employee health that focuses resources on exposure controls by describing how a risk needs to be managed. Information on control banding is available at http://www.cdc.gov/niosh/topics/ctrlbanding/. This approach can be applied in situations where OELs have not been established or can be used to supplement the OELs, when available.

Silica (Quartz and Cristobalite)

Silica or silicon dioxide occurs in a crystalline or noncrystalline (amorphous) form. In crystalline silica, the silicon dioxide molecules are oriented in a fixed pattern versus the random arrangement of the amorphous form. The more common crystalline forms in workplace environments are quartz and cristobalite, and to a lesser extent, tridymite. Occupational exposures to respirable crystalline silica (quartz and cristobalite) have been associated with silicosis, lung cancer, pulmonary tuberculosis, and airway diseases.

Silicosis is a fibrotic disease of the lung caused by the deposition of fine crystalline silica particles in the lungs. It is the disease most often associated with exposure to respirable crystalline silica. This lung disease is caused by the inhalation and deposition of crystalline silica particles that are 10 μm or less in diameter. Particles 10 μm or below are considered respirable particles and classified as having the potential to reach the lower portions of the human lung (alveolar region). Although particle sizes 10 μm and below are considered respirable, some of these particles can be deposited before they reach the alveolar region [Hinds 1999]. Symptoms of silicosis usually develop insidiously, with cough, shortness of breath, chest pain, weakness, wheezing, and nonspecific chest illnesses. Silicosis usually occurs after years of exposure (chronic), but may appear in a shorter period of time (acute) if exposure concentrations are very high. Acute silicosis is typically associated with a history of high exposures from tasks that produce small particles of airborne dust with a high silica content [NIOSH 1986]. Even though the carcinogenicity of crystalline silica in humans has been strongly debated in the scientific community, IARC in 1996 concluded that there was "sufficient evidence in humans for the carcinogenicity of inhaled crystalline silica in the form of quartz or cristobalite from occupational sources [IARC 1997]." A NIOSH publication also lists several other serious diseases from occupational exposure to crystalline silica. These include lung cancer and noncarcinogenic disorders including immunologic disorders and autoimmune diseases, rheumatoid arthritis, renal diseases, and an increased risk of developing tuberculosis after exposure to the infectious agent [NIOSH 2002].

When proper practices are not followed or controls are not maintained, respirable crystalline silica exposures can exceed the NIOSH REL, the ACGIH TLV, or the OSHA PEL. NIOSH recommends an exposure limit of 0.05 mg/m³, TWA for up to a 10-hour work day to reduce the risk of developing silicosis, lung cancer, and other adverse health effects [NIOSH 2005]. The ACGIH TLV for quartz is 0.025 mg/m³, TWA for up to an 8-hour work day [ACGIH 2009].

The current OSHA PEL for respirable dust containing crystalline silica (quartz) for the construction industry is measured by impinger sampling. The PEL is expressed in mppcf and is calculated using the following formula [29 CFR 1926.55]:

$$\text{Respirable PEL} = \frac{250 \text{ mppcf}}{\% \text{ Silica} + 5}$$

Since the PELs were adopted, the impinger sampling method has been rendered obsolete by gravimetric sampling [OSHA 1996]. OSHA is not aware of any government agencies or employers in this country that are currently using impinger sampling to assess worker exposure to dust containing crystalline silica, and impinger samples are generally recognized as less reliable than gravimetric samples. OSHA currently instructs its compliance officers to apply a conversion factor of 0.1 mg/m³ per mppcf when converting between gravimetric sampling and the particle count standard when characterizing construction operation exposures [OSHA 2001]. Virginia OSHA uses the conversion factor to calculate mppcf and ultimately compare to the calculated construction PEL [VDLI 2010]. Therefore, in this report, respirable dust concentrations are presented in mppcf.

Isocyanates (including MDI)

Diisocyanates are a group of highly reactive, low-molecular-weight aromatic and aliphatic compounds, characterized by two isocyanate functional groups (N=C=O). The most common diisocyanates include the aliphatic compounds, hexamethylene diisocyanate and isophorone diisocyanate, and the aromatic compounds, toluene diisocyanate and MDI. Monomeric and polymeric diisocyanates are widely used in the production of polyurethane materials such as foams, adhesives, resins, elastomers, binders, and coatings. In industry, polyurethane is synthesized via a polymer chemistry reaction between polyisocyanates and polyols.

Exposure to isocyanates can be irritating to the skin, mucous membranes, eyes, and respiratory tract [NIOSH 1978, 2005]. The most frequent respiratory effect associated with isocyanate exposure is asthma due to sensitization [Markowitz 2005; NIOSH 2005]. Contact dermatitis (both irritant and allergic forms) is less common and can result in symptoms such as rash, erythema, and itching [Goossens et al. 2002]. An employee with isocyanate-induced asthma exhibits the traditional symptoms of acute airway obstruction such as coughing, wheezing, shortness of breath, tightness in the chest, and nocturnal awakening [NIOSH 1978, 1986]. Isocyanate-induced asthma occurs with variable latency following the initial exposure, although characteristically the asthma develops within 2 years of exposure [Markowitz 2005]. The asthmatic reaction may occur minutes after exposure (immediate onset) and/or several hours after exposure (delayed onset) [Chan-Yeung and Lam 1986; NIOSH 1986]. After sensitization, any exposure, even to levels below OELs, can produce an asthmatic response that may be life threatening [NIOSH 1978, 1996, 2006].

Monomeric, polymeric, and prepolymeric isocyanates appear to be capable of producing respiratory sensitization in exposed employees [Harries et al. 1979; Berlin et al. 1981; Woolrich 1982; Mobay Corporation 1983, 1991; Zammit-Tabona et al. 1983; Chang and Karol 1984; Nielsen et al. 1985; Alexandersson et al. 1986; Seguin et al. 1987; Mapp et al. 1988; Liss et al. 1988; Keskinen et al. 1988; Cartier et al. 1989; Vandenplas et al. 1992a,b; Baur et al. 1994]. Several animal studies have shown that dermal exposure to diisocyanates may also produce respiratory sensitization [Karol et al. 1981; Erjefalt and Persson 1992; Bickis 1994; Rattray et al. 1994; Herrick 2002]. Employees exposed to isocyanates primarily through the dermal route have developed respiratory sensitization and occupational asthma in addition to skin sensitization (allergic contact dermatitis) [Bello 2007].

Diagnosis of isocyanate-induced asthma requires a thorough occupational history. As with other asthmatic conditions, pulmonary function tests may be within normal limits between asthmatic episodes. The prevalence of diisocyanate-induced asthma in exposed workers is believed to be 5%–10% [Chan-Yeung and Malo 1995; Bernstein 1996]. The only effective intervention for employees with isocyanate-induced asthma is cessation of all isocyanate exposure. This can be accomplished by removing the employee from the work environment where isocyanate exposure occurs.

The current OELs for the different isocyanates are provided in Table 1. Most of the OELs apply to specific diisocyanates. However, the UK HSE has developed a standard based on the concentration of TRIG in a volume of air [Silk and Hardy 1983]. TRIG is a measurement of the concentration of isocyanate functional groups (N=C=O) in a sample of air. Airborne TRIG concentrations can be determined using NIOSH Method 5525 [NIOSH 2009].

References

ACGIH [2009]. 2009 TLVs® and BEIs®: threshold limit values for chemical substances and physical agents and biological exposure indices. Cincinnati, OH: American Conference of Governmental Industrial Hygienists.

Table A1. Current OELs ($\mu g/m^3$) for isocyanates

	OSHA PEL [29 CFR 1910.1000]		NIOSH REL [NIOSH 2005]		ACGIH TLV [ACGIH 2009]		UK HSE [HSE 2005]	
	8-hr TWA	Ceiling	10-hr TWA	10-min ceiling	8-hr TWA	15-min STEL	8-hr TWA	10-min ceiling
TDI*		140			36	140		
MDI		240	50	200	51			
HDI†			35	140	34			
IPDI‡			45	180	45			
TRIG							20	70

* toluene diisocyanate
† hexamethylene diisocyanate
‡ isophorone diisocyanate

AIHA [2009]. AIHA 2009 Emergency response planning guidelines (ERPG) & workplace environmental exposure levels (WEEL) handbook. Fairfax, VA: American Industrial Hygiene Association.

Alexandersson R, Gustafsson P, Hedenstierna G, Rosen G [1986]. Exposure to naphthalene-diisocyanate in a rubber plant: symptoms and lung function. Arch Environ Health 41(2):85–89.

Baur X, Marek W, Ammon J, Czuppon AB, Marczynski B, Raulf-Heimsoth M, Roemmelt H, Fruhmann G [1994]. Respiratory and other hazards of isocyanates. Int Arch Occup Environ Health 66(3):141–152.

Bello D, Herrick CA, Smith TJ, Woskie SR, Streicher RP, Cullen MR, Liu Y, Redlich CA [2007]. Skin exposure to isocyanates: reasons for concern. Environ Health Perspect 115(3):328–335.

Berlin L, Hjortsberg U, Wass U [1981]. Life-threatening pulmonary reaction to car paint containing a prepolymerized isocyanate. Scand J Work Environ Health 7(4):310–312.

Bernstein JA [1996]. Overview of diisocyanate occupational asthma. Toxicology 111(1-3):181–189.

Bickis U [1994]. Investigation of dermally induced airway hyperreactivity to toluene diisocyanate in guinea pigs. Ph.D. Dissertation, Department of Pharmacology and Toxicology, Queens University, Kingston, Ontario, Canada.

Cartier A, Grammar L, Malo JL, Lagier F, Ghezzo H, Harris K, Patterson R [1989]. Specific serum antibodies against isocyanates: association with occupational asthma. J Allergy Clin Immunol 84(4 Pt 1):507–514.

CFR. Code of Federal Regulations. Washington, DC: U.S. Government Printing Office, Office of the Federal Register.

Chan-Yeung M, Lam S [1986]. Occupational asthma. Am Rev Respir Dis 133(4):686–703.

Chan-Yeung M, Malo JL [1995]. Occupational asthma. N Engl J Med 333(2):107–112.

Chang KC, Karol MH [1984]. Diphenylmethane diisocyanate (MDI)-induced asthma: evaluation of immunologic responses and application of an animal model of isocyanate sensitivity. Clin Allergy 14(4):329–339.

Erjefalt I, Persson CGA [1992]. Increased sensitivity to toluene diisocyanate (TDI) in airways previously exposed to low doses of TDI. Clin Exp Allergy 22(9):854–862.

Goossens A, Detienne T, Bruze M [2002]. Occupational contact dermatitis caused by isocyanates. Contact Dermatitis 47(5):304–308.

Harries M, Burge S, Samson M, Taylor A, Pepys J [1979]. Isocyanate asthma: respiratory symptoms due to 1,5-naphthylene di-isocyanate. Thorax 34(6):762–766.

Herrick CA, Xu L, Wisnewski AV, Das J, Redlich CA, Bottomly K [2002]. A novel mouse model of diisocyanate-induced asthma showing allergic-type inflammation in the lung after inhaled antigen challenge. J Allergy Clin Immunol 109(5):873–878.

Hinds WC [1999]. Aerosol technology: properties, behavior, and measurement of airborne particles. 2nd ed. New York: John Wiley & Sons, Inc., pp. 239–242.

HSE [2005]. Workplace exposure limits, EH40/2005. Sudbury, England: Health and Safety Executive, HSE Books.

IARC [1997]. IARC monographs on the evaluation of carcinogenic risks to humans: silica, some silicates, coal dust and para-aramid fibrils. Vol. 68. Lyon, France: World Health Organization, International Agency for Research on Cancer.

Karol MH, Hauth BA, Riley EJ, Magreni CM [1981]. Dermal contact with toluene diisocyanate (TDI) produces respiratory tract hypersensitivity in guinea pigs. Toxicol Appl Pharmacol 58(2):221–230.

Keskinen H, Tupasela O, Tiikkainen U, Nordman H [1988]. Experiences of specific IgE in asthma due to diisocyanates. Clin Allergy 18(6):597–604.

Liss GM, Bernstein DI, Moller DR, Gallagher JS, Stephenson RL, Bernstein IL [1988]. Pulmonary and immunologic evaluation of foundry workers exposed to methylene diphenyldiisocyanate (MDI). J Allergy Clin Immunol 82(1):55–61.

Mapp CE, Chiesura-Corona P, DeMarzo N, Fabbri L [1988]. Persistent asthma due to isocyanates. Am Rev Resp Dis 137(6):1326–1329.

Markowitz S [2005]. Chemicals in the plastics, synthetic textiles, and rubber industries. In: Rosenstock L, Cullen M, Brodkin C, Redlich C, eds. Textbook of clinical occupational and environmental medicine, 2nd ed. Philadelphia: Elsevier Saunders Publishers, pp. 1021–1022.

Mobay Corporation [1983]. Health & safety information for MDI, diphenylmethane diisocyanate, monomeric, polymeric, modified. Pittsburgh, PA: Mobay Corporation.

Mobay Corporation [1991]. Hexamethylene diisocyanate based polyisocyanates, health and safety information. Pittsburgh, PA: Mobay Corporation.

Nielsen J, Sungo C, Winroth G, Hallberg T, Skerfving S [1985]. Systemic reactions associated with polyisocyanate exposure. Scand J Work Environ Health 11(1):51–54.

NIOSH [1978]. Criteria for a recommended standard: occupational exposure to diisocyanates. By Soucek S. Cincinnati, OH: U.S. Dept. of Health, Education, and Welfare, Center for Disease Control, National Institute for Occupational Safety and Health, DHEW (NIOSH) Publication No. 78-215.

NIOSH [1986]. Occupational respiratory diseases. Merchant JA, Boehlecke BA, Taylor G, Pickett-Harner M. Cincinnati, OH: U.S. Department of Health and Human Services, Centers for Disease Control, National Institute for Occupational Safety and Health, DHHS (NIOSH) Publication No. 86-102.

NIOSH [1996]. NIOSH alert: preventing asthma and death from diisocyanate exposure. Cincinnati, OH: U.S. Dept. of Health and Human Services, Centers for Disease Control, National Institute for Occupational Safety and Health, DHHS (NIOSH) Publication No. 96-111.

NIOSH [2002]. NIOSH Hazard Review: health effects of occupational exposure to respirable silica. By Rice FL. Cincinnati, OH: U.S. Department of Health and Human Services, Centers for Disease Control and Prevention, National Institute for Occupational Safety and Health, DHHS (NIOSH) Publication No. 2002-129.

NIOSH [2005]. NIOSH pocket guide to chemical hazards. Cincinnati, OH: U.S. Department of Health and Human Services, Centers for Disease Control and Prevention, National Institute for Occupational Safety and Health, DHHS (NIOSH) Publication No. 2005-149. [http://www.cdc.gov/niosh/npg/]. Date accessed: December 2009.

NIOSH [2006]. NIOSH alert: preventing asthma and death from MDI exposure during spray-on truck bed liner and related applications. Cincinnati, OH: U.S. Dept. of Health and Human Services, Centers for Disease Control, National Institute for Occupational Safety and Health, DHHS (NIOSH) Publication No. 2006-149.

NIOSH [2009]. NIOSH manual of analytical methods (NMAM®). 4th ed. Schlecht PC, O'Connor PF, eds. Cincinnati, OH: U.S. Department of Health and Human Services, Centers for Disease Control and

Prevention, National Institute for Occupational Safety and Health, DHHS (NIOSH) Publication 94-113 (August, 1994); 1st Supplement Publication 96-135, 2nd Supplement Publication 98-119; 3rd Supplement 2003-154. [http://www.cdc.gov/niosh/docs/2003-154/].

OSHA [1996]. Memorandum for regional administrators from: Joseph A. Dear. Subject: special emphasis program (SEP) for silicosis. May 2, 1996. Appendix F: Permissible Exposure Limits for Construction. [http://www.osha.gov/dcsp/ote/trng-materials/silicosis/specialemphasismemo.html]. Date accessed: December 31, 2007.

OSHA [2001]. Memorandum for regional administrators and silica coordinators from: Richard E. Fairfax Director, Directorate of Compliance Programs. Subject: transmission of NIOSH recommended conversion factor for silica sample results and favorable appellate court decision on silica sampling. September 4, 2001.

Rattray NJ, Bothman PA, Hext PM, Woodcock DR, Fielding I, Dearman RJ, Kimber I [1994]. Induction of respiratory hypersensitivity to diphenylmethane-4,4'-diisocyanate (MDI) in guinea pigs. Influence of route of exposure. Toxicol 88(1-3):15–30.

Seguin P, Allard A, Cartier A, Malo JL [1987]. Prevalence of occupational asthma in spray painters exposed to several types of isocyanates, including polymethylene polyphenyl isocyanate. J Occup Med 29(4):340–344.

Silk SJ, Hardy HL [1983]. Control limits for isocyanates. Ann Occup Hyg 27(4):333–339.

Vandenplas O, Cartier A, Lesage J, Perrault G, Grammar LC, Malo JL [1992a]. Occupational asthma caused by a prepolymer but not the monomer of toluene diisocyanate (TDI). J Allergy Clin Immunol 89(6):1183–1188.

VDLI [2010]. Telephone conversation on May 27, 2010, between the Virginia Department of Labor and Industry and R. McCleery of the Division of Surveillance, Hazard Evaluations and Field Studies, National Institute for Occupational Safety and Health, Centers for Disease Control and Prevention, U.S. Department of Health and Human Services.

Vandenplas O, Cartier A, Lesage J, Cloutier Y, Perrault G, Grammar LC, Shaughnessy MA, Malo JL [1992b]. Prepolymers of hexamethylene diisocyanate as a cause of occupational asthma. J Allergy Clin Immunol 91(4):850–861.

Woolrich PF [1982]. Toxicology, industrial hygiene and medical control of TDI, MDI, and PMPPI. Am Ind Hyg Assoc J 43(2):89–98.

Zammit-Tabona M, Sherkin M, Kijek K, Chan H, Chan-Yeung M [1983]. Asthma caused by diphenylmethane diisocyanate in foundry workers. Am Rev Resp Dis 128(2):226–230.

Acknowledgments and
Availability of Report

The Hazard Evaluations and Technical Assistance Branch (HETAB) of the National Institute for Occupational Safety and Health (NIOSH) conducts field investigations of possible health hazards in the workplace. These investigations are conducted under the authority of Section 20(a)(6) of the Occupational Safety and Health Act of 1970, 29 U.S.C. 669(a)(6) which authorizes the Secretary of Health and Human Services, following a written request from any employer or authorized representative of employees, to determine whether any substance normally found in the place of employment has potentially toxic effects in such concentrations as used or found. HETAB also provides, upon request, technical and consultative assistance to federal, state, and local agencies; labor; industry; and other groups or individuals to control occupational health hazards and to prevent related trauma and disease.

The findings and conclusions in this report are those of the authors and do not necessarily represent the views of NIOSH. Mention of any company or product does not constitute endorsement by NIOSH. In addition, citations to websites external to NIOSH do not constitute NIOSH endorsement of the sponsoring organization or their programs or products. Furthermore, NIOSH is not responsible for the content of these websites. All Web addresses referenced in this document were accessible as of the publication date.

This report was prepared by Chandran Achutan and Ayodele Adebayo of HETAB, Division of Surveillance, Hazard Evaluations and Field Studies and Fariba Nourian of the Division of Applied Research and Technology (DART). Industrial hygiene field assistance was provided by SeungHee Jang. Analytical support was provided by Kathleen Ernst and Robert Streicher of DART, and Bureau Veritas, Michigan. Health communication assistance was provided by Stefanie Evans. Editorial assistance was provided by Ellen Galloway. Desktop publishing was performed by Robin Smith.

Copies of this report have been sent to employee and management representatives at Aduddell Restoration and Waterproofing Company and the Occupational Safety and Health Administration Regional Office. This report is not copyrighted and may be freely reproduced. The report may be viewed and printed from the following internet address: http://www.cdc.gov/niosh/hhe. Copies may be purchased from the National Technical Information Service at 5825 Port Royal Road, Springfield, Virginia 22161.

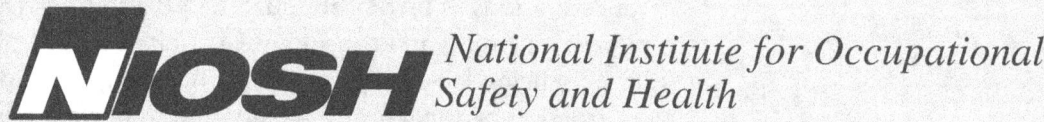 National Institute for Occupational Safety and Health

Delivering on the Nation's promise: Safety and health at work for all people through research and prevention.

To receive NIOSH documents or information about occupational safety and health topics, contact NIOSH at:

1-800-CDC-INFO (1-800-232-4636)

TTY: 1-888-232-6348

E-mail: cdcinfo@cdc.gov

or visit the NIOSH web site at: **www.cdc.gov/niosh.**

For a monthly update on news at NIOSH, subscribe to NIOSH eNews by visiting **www.cdc.gov/niosh/eNews.**

SAFER • HEALTHIER • PEOPLE™